1 Top 10 Health Benefits Of Being Vegetarian

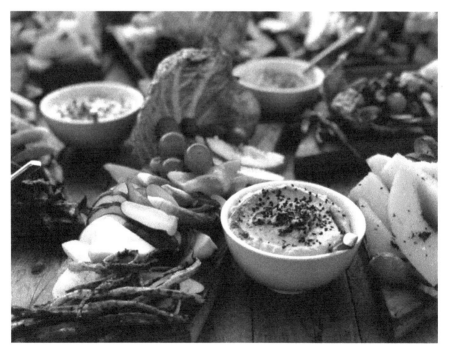

Top 10 Health Benefits Of Being Vegetarian

What is vegetarianism?

Vegetarianism is the practice of abstaining from the consumption of animal products including red meat, fish or other seafood, poultry, the flesh of animal or by-products of animal slaughter. A vegetarian diet includes grains, fruits, vegetables, pulses, nuts, seeds, and with, or without, the use of dairy products and eggs.

There are different types of vegetarians:

- **Lacto-vegetarians** exclude animal products and eggs but eat dairy products.

- **Lacto-ovo-vegetarians** exclude animal products but eat both dairy products and eggs.

- **Jain vegetarians** exclude animal products, eggs, or anything that grows underground including potatoes, onions, and garlic but eat dairy products.

- **Buddhist Vegetarians** exclude animal products and vegetables in the allium family (which have the characteristic aroma of onion and garlic): onion, garlic, chives, scallions, leeks, or shallots but eat dairy products.

- **Vegans** exclude any products derived from animals – no meat, fish, dairy or eggs.

Below are the Top 10 Health benefits of being vegetarian:

1. Slows the Aging Process, Increases Lifespan

Vegetarian organic plant-based diet is mainly rich in vitamins and minerals, antioxidants, phytonutrients and fiber which in turn strengthens the immune system and flushes out toxin from the body, prevent chemical build up in the body slows down the aging process. Additionally, a vegetarian diet can prevent many chronic diseases thus facilitating more healthy years and a longer lifespan.

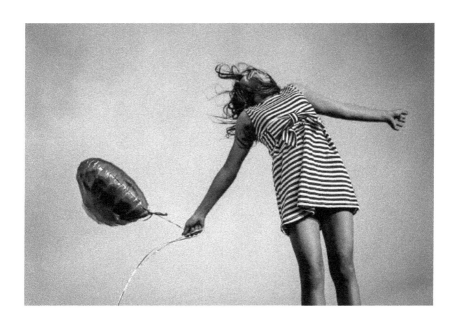

2. Less Toxicity

Toxins such as pesticides, antibiotics, hormones are all fat-soluble, they concentrate in the fatty flesh of the animals. Non-Vegetarian foods can harbor contaminants such viruses and parasites such as toxoplasmosis parasites, Trichinella spiralis, salmonella, and other worms. Food-borne illnesses, bacteria, and chemical toxins are more common in commercial meat, seafood, and poultry when compared with organic plant-based foods.

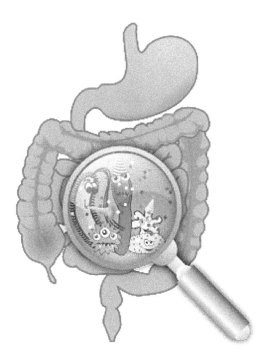

3. Improves metabolism

Fiber is necessary for proper digestion and fruits and vegetables contain high fiber content. Vegetarian food is easy to digest and helps in fast elimination of toxins and other chemicals from the body keeping the body metabolism in a good state. RMR (resting metabolic rate) in people with a vegetarian diet is higher than omnivores which means vegetarians speedily burn fats.

4. Maintains Healthy Body Weight

Typically, Vegetarians weigh less. Vegetarians tend to have a lower body mass index (a measure of body fat) than meat eaters'. This may be because a vegetarian diet typically comprised of fewer calories and high in fiber-rich such as fruits, and vegetables, grains, legumes, nuts and seeds that are more filling, lower in fat and less calorie dense. This might be the main reason why more and more people today are opting vegetarianism in their life.

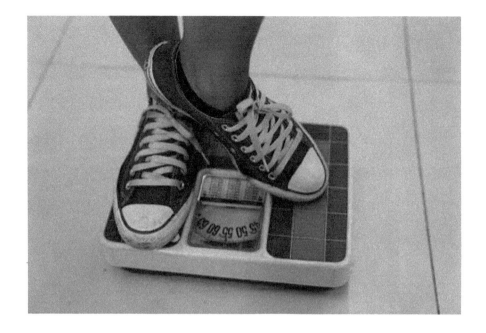

5. Reduces Risk of Diabetes

As per a study, diabetes is more frequently occurs in Non-vegetarians almost twice as often as in vegetarians. Vegetarian diet provides greater protection against diabetes. A healthy vegetarian diet is easy to absorb, contains less fatty acids and is nutritious. Vegetarian diets have been shown to be beneficial for people with Type 2 diabetes where weight loss is often the most effective way to manage the condition.

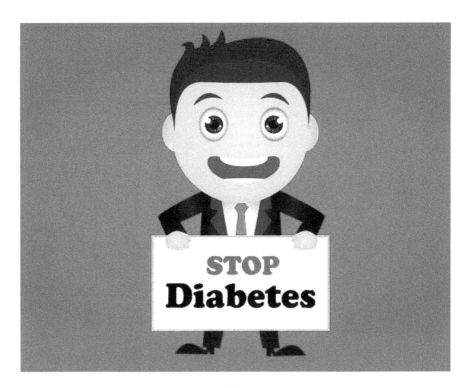

6. Reduces Risk of Cataract

Though it cannot be confirmed that eating meat causes cataract development, but many studies have revealed that decreases in meat consumption as part of a daily diet decreases the risk for cataracts. Researchers suggest that the overall lifestyle of vegetarians contribute to the decreased risk of cataract and vegetarians enjoy less incidence of cataract development.

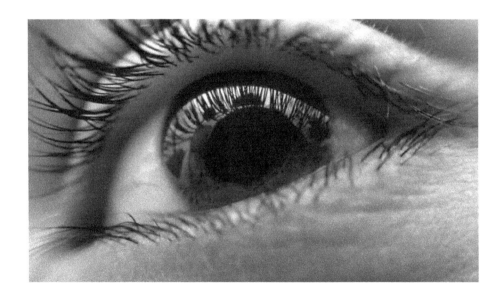

7. Reduces Risk of Cancer

Red meat and processed meat consumption are directly associated with an increase in the risk of colorectal cancer. Regularly consuming is strongly associated with a reduced risk of some cancers. There is evidence that vegetarians have a statistically significant lower rate of cancer than those who consumed meat regularly. The vegetarian diet contains fruits and vegetables that are high in antioxidants which protect against cancer. Reducing your risk of cancer is another great reason to opt for vegetarianism.

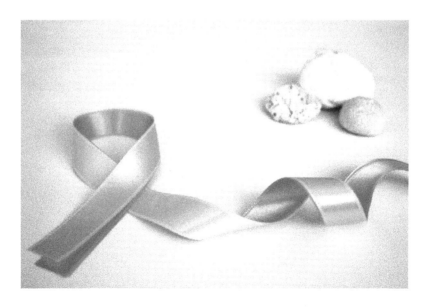

8. Reduces Risk of Heart Disease

Vegetarian diets are rich in fiber, anti-oxidants, and phytonutrients, which are known to reduce oxidative stress and inflammation which may support a significantly reduced the risk of heart disease. Also, Vegetarian diets are lower in saturated fat and cholesterol in comparison to meat-based diets that are often high in cholesterol, fat and environmental pollutants. Vegetarians have 40 percent less risk of death from cardiovascular disease than non-vegetarians.

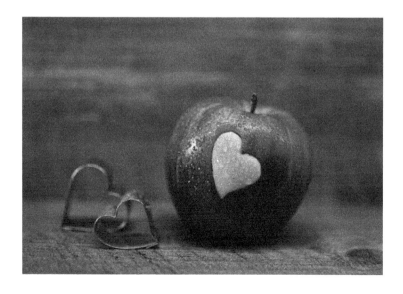

9. Gives More Energy

Vegetarians are tending to be more energetic and happy. Meat-based diet is often high in fat and protein making them difficult to digest while vegetarians have a higher consumption of carbohydrates in the form of whole grain. Carbohydrates digest easily and give energy instantly. Carbohydrates increase serotonin levels, which is mood-boosting neurotransmitter which increases the brain's serotonin levels called happiness hormones which keep you happy all day.

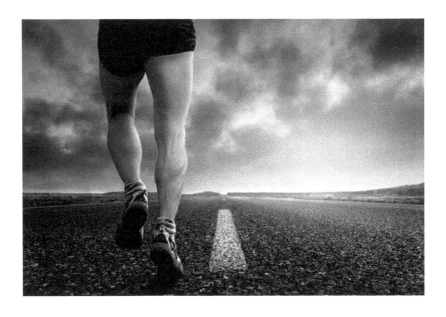

10. Lowers Cholesterol Levels

Vegetarian diet is much low in cholesterol while animal products are very high in cholesterol. High levels of low-density lipoprotein (LDL) cholesterol (bad cholesterol) have been linked with an increased risk of coronary heart disease (CHD).

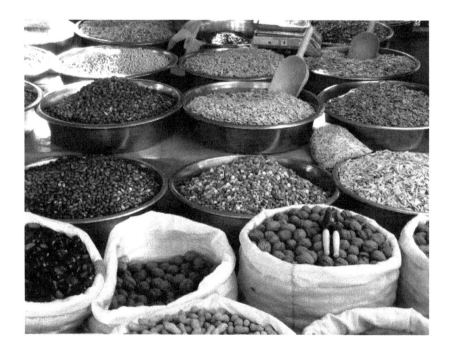

Vegetarian Diet Is Associated with lower cholesterol levels. This may be due to the Vegetarians have reduced intake of saturated fat, and an increased intake of organic plant-based foods, like fruits, vegetables, whole grains, legumes, seeds, and nuts, which are naturally rich in soluble fiber, soy protein, and plant sterols. Although cholesterol is an essential component of each human cell, there is no need to take cholesterol from an external source as the body can make all the cholesterol it needs from Vegetarian foods.

Conclusion

Along with healthy organic vegetarian diet, there are many factors that attribute to a healthy and long lifespan, some other lifestyles need to pay attention like quitting smoking and drinking. Being on a vegetarian diet doesn't mean you opt for less healthy food options, such as refined grains, which could increase the risk of heart disease. One should follow plant-based diets that are high in fiber, whole grains, vegetables, legumes, seeds and nuts that are lower in fat, more filling, healthy and nutritious.

2 10 Reasons You Should Eat More Protein Every Day

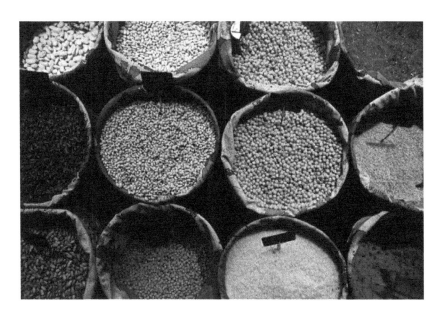

10 Reasons You Should Eat More Protein Every Day

What is Protein?

Proteins are essential macronutrients, consisting of one or more long chain of amino acid which is the essential part of all living organisms, especially as the building blocks of body tissue such as muscle, hair, bones, nails, etc.

Daily Recommended Protein Amount

Recommended Dietary Allowances (RDA), the daily dietary intake level of a nutrient considered sufficient to meet your basic nutritional requirements. RDA for protein is 0.8 grams of protein per kilogram of body weight.

RDA is shown below for males and females aged 19-70 years:

Male: 56 g/day

Female: 46 g/day

Below are the 10 Reasons You Should Eat More Protein Every Day:

1. Anti-Aging

Wrinkles are primarily caused by sun damage and loss of the proteins collagen and elastin. As we grow older our body inevitably loses muscle mass. One of the easiest ways to improve your muscle mass and to keep your body healthy is to follow a protein-rich diet which accelerates the healing and nourishing skin. Whey protein is good for anti-aging nutrition it contains branch chain amino acids which heal and nourish skin and prevent aging signs.

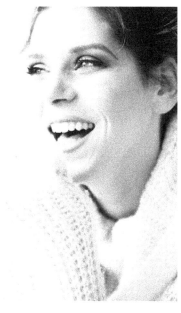

2. Speeds Up Recovery From Injury

Protein is an important building block of body tissues, including muscle. Protein can help the body repair after it has been injured. It speeds up the recovery process. Protein digests into the amino acids which are required to repair damaged muscles, the body needs a steady stream of amino acids to promote healing. Protein helps to rebuild any lost muscle. Body needs extra protein post-injury. The protein-rich diet allows the body to produce new collagen and elastin to help keep tendons and ligaments strong.

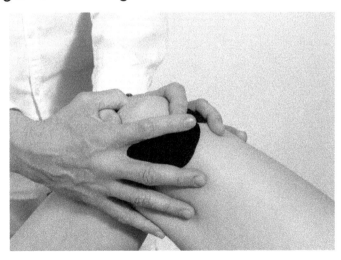

3. Boost Muscle Mass

Protein is the building block of muscles. Eating adequate amounts of protein promotes muscle growth and helps in maintaining muscle mass. To gain muscle mass one should do exercise and strength training along with high rich protein diet. Also, the constant supply of Protein throughout the day is essential for optimum muscle growth.

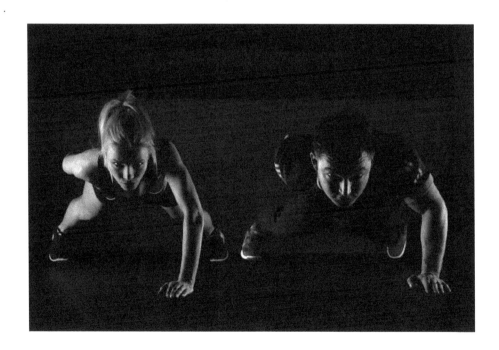

4. Healthy Skin

Protein is a building block of skin tissue. It is great for the general health of skin and for its ability to repair itself. Proteins are broken down into amino acids, for the body's constant reconstruction job. Amino acids help to construct collagen, create lubricating ceramide in the skin which keeps the skin healthy. It also repairs the skin-damaging done by the sun and environmental irritants.

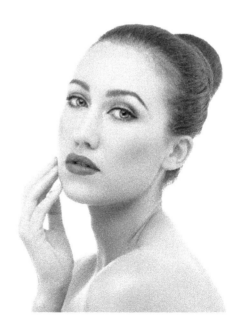

5. Reduces Appetite, Increases Satiety

Protein helps you stay full for longer with less food. Eating a high-protein diet can boost the release of a hunger-suppressing hormone peptide. That means you don't get cravings, and it means you control your hunger. Protein also reduces levels of appetite-spiking hormone ghrelin so you don't get massive cravings at nights. It can make you eat fewer calories automatically.

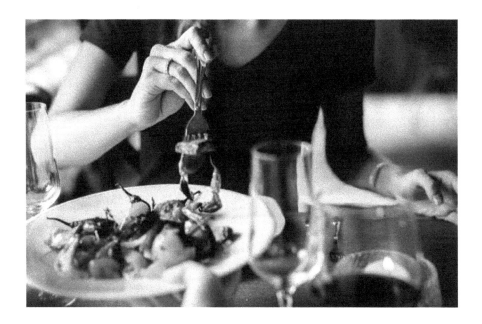

6. Burns More Calories

When you replace some of carbs and fat with protein in your diet you actually burn more calories as protein gives a boost to your metabolism. This is because our body needs some calories for the purpose of digesting and metabolizing the food. The number of calories required to burn protein into fuel is much higher than fats and carbs, it means your body will burn way more calories over the course of the day. This way your metabolism will be more efficient and you lose more weight.

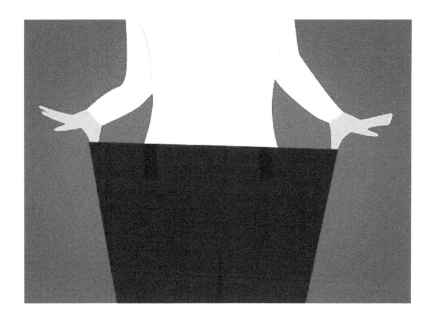

7. Controls Diabetes

A Diet high in protein and low in carbohydrates may help Type 2 diabetes patients improve their blood sugar levels. Protein is broken down into glucose less efficiently than carbohydrate and, as a result, takes longer to reach the bloodstream, cause insulin to release gradually, helping the body maintain healthy glucose levels.

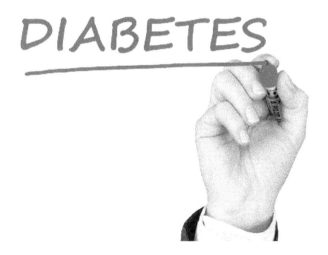

8. Lowers Blood Pressure

Short-term clinical trials suggest that dietary protein lowers blood pressure. High-protein diets might reduce the risk of cardiovascular disease by lowering blood pressure. Increasing protein intake may actually help lower systolic blood pressure. Higher protein diets also characterized by higher fiber intakes lead to a 59% reduction in High Blood Pressure risk.

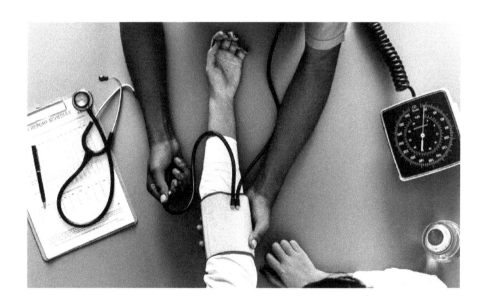

9. Healthy Bones

Osteoporosis is a huge issue especially for women after menopause. Improving bone health is an important component of treating and preventing osteoporosis. Protein represents key nutrients for bone health. Protein is crucial for the body's ability to absorb calcium and grow bones strong. People who eat more protein tend to have a lower risk of osteoporosis and fractures and maintain better bone mass as they age.

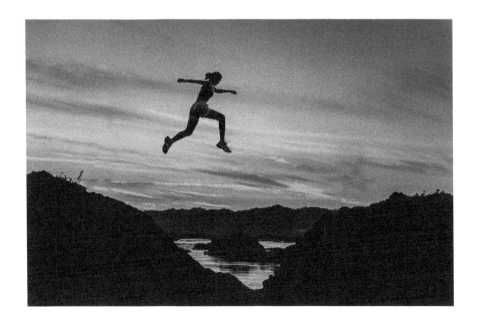

10. Healthy Hair

Eating enough protein is important for healthy and strong hair. Protein promotes hair growth because hair follicles are made of mostly protein. Protein-rich diet helps the body to produce keratin, which is fundamental to the hair structure. When keratin weakens, hair strands become dry and brittle. One should eat high protein and iron rich diet to prevent hair loss.

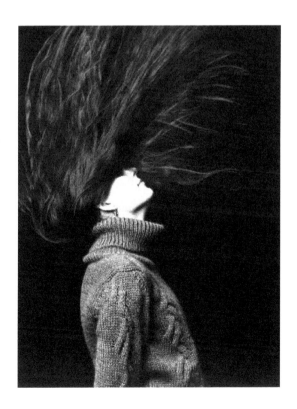

Conclusion

Protein is the basic requirement of the body for repairing, making enzymes, hormones, and other body chemicals. Protein intake should definitely be increased for a healthy life but anything in excess is harmful to health. Too much protein can be harmful to people with kidney disease. Just because protein helps in faster weight lose it is never be advised to completely replace carbs and fats with protein in your diet. Excess of protein may cause bloating, gas, stomach cramps and diarrhea when a lot of protein is fermented in the colon, or if you're low in digestive acids and enzymes.

3 10 High Protein Sources For Vegetarians

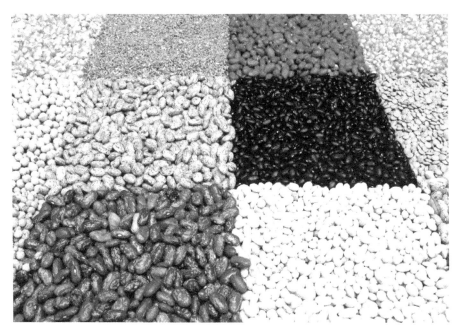

10 High Protein Sources For Vegetarians

Protein is the building blocks of body tissue such as muscle, hair, bones, nails. Protein deficiency is a very common concern about vegetarian diets. However, animal protein is associated with many of the degenerative diseases while vegetable protein isn't.

Sufficient protein intake is a must for all human beings despite the age or gender as higher-protein diets boost muscle mass, faster recovery from injury, healthy skin and weight loss.

Below are the 10 High Protein Sources For Vegetarians:

1. Whey Of Cottage Cheese

The liquid portion of the cottage cheese making process is called whey. Whey is a great source of protein for vegetarians. Whey protein can help increase fat loss while providing protein and amino acids, which serve as building blocks for increased muscle growth. You can easily make cottage cheese at home by adding 2 tablespoon lemon juice to 200 ml boiling milk. The acidity of lemon juice will coagulate the milk. Separate the solid and liquid portion. The solid part is the cottage cheese and the remaining liquid is your whey.

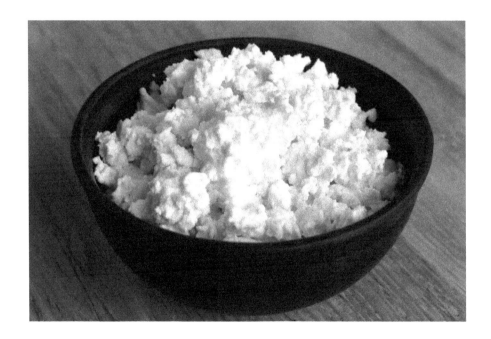

2. Peanuts

Peanuts have more protein than any other nuts. In addition, they are loaded with healthful nutrients, such as antioxidants, fiber, iron, and magnesium. Fats in peanuts are healthful fats, which can help lower bad LDL cholesterol and may improve heart health.

100 grams of peanuts contain 26 grams of protein.

Peanuts recipes: Sabudana Khichdi, Crunchy Peanut Chocolate Bars, Roasted Spicy Peanuts.

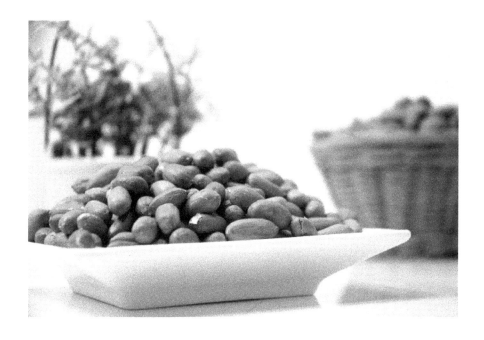

3. Kidney Beans

Kidney beans are low in fats, are excellent sources of protein. They are also a good source of fiber, vitamins, and minerals. Kidney beans contain all nine-amino acid. They are a good source of lysine, an amino acid which is usually lack in other plant-based protein sources, such as grains.

100 grams of kidney beans contain 24 grams of protein.

Kidney Beans recipes: Mexican Bean Soup, Rajma (Kidney Bean Curry), Vegetarian chili tacos.

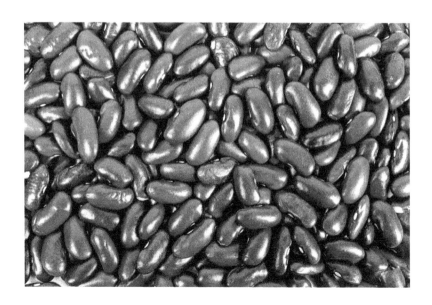

4. Oats

Oats contain more protein than most grains. Oat protein is nearly equivalent in quality to soy protein, which is equal to meat, milk and egg protein as per WHO. Oats are one of the easy ways to add protein to your diet.

100 grams of the hull-less oat kernels contain 12-24 grams of protein, the highest among cereals.

Oats recipes: Vegetable Oats Cutlets, Oatmeal Cookies, Oats Upma.

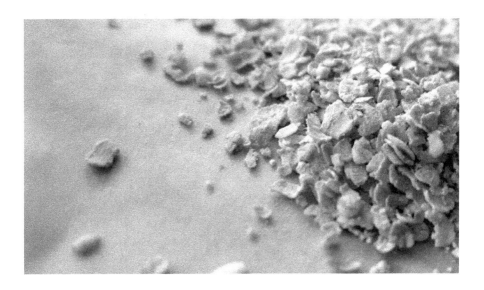

5. Almonds

Almonds are an excellent source of protein. These are also rich in fiber and vitamin E, which is great for the skin. One should eat at least 10 almonds every day, not only for protein but for its other health benefits too. It is advised to eat overnight soaked almonds because it reduces the number of tannins and acids present in the skin of the almond, which can inhibit nutrient uptake by the body.

100 grams of almonds contain 21 grams of protein.

Almonds recipes: Almond Cake, Dry Fruits Milk Shake, Almond Cookies.

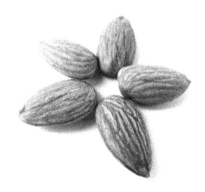

6. Chickpeas

Chickpeas are a great source of plant-based protein. There are plenty of chickpeas recipes available which can satisfy your taste bud as well as fulfill your daily protein requirement.

100 grams of chickpeas contain 19 grams of protein.

Chickpeas recipes: Hummus spread, Falafel, Indian Chana masala.

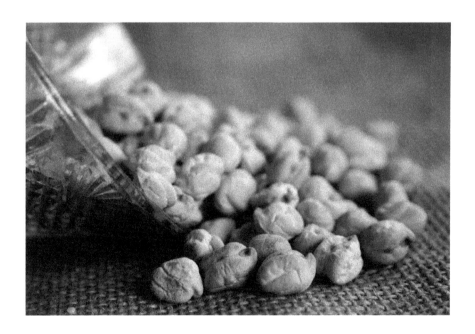

7. Amaranth

Amaranth is a protein powerhouse. Amaranth is high in protein and lysine, an amino acid found in low quantities in other grains. Amaranth grain is free of gluten, which makes it a viable grain for people with gluten intolerance. Amaranth is rich in fiber and also a good source of manganese, magnesium, vitamin B6, phosphorus and iron.

100 grams of amaranth contains 14 grams of protein.

Amaranth recipes: Amaranth and Almond Ladoo, Amaranth cutlets, Amaranth Flour, and Raisin Cookies.

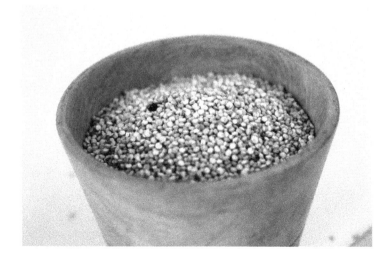

8. Greek Yogurt

Greek yogurt is higher in protein than regular yogurt. Greek yogurt is strained three times, so most of the whey is removed. It also has less carbohydrate than regular yogurt, since some of the whey is removed. Because Greek yogurt is more concentrated, it has more protein than regular yogurt.

100 grams of Greek yogurt contains 10 grams of protein.

Greek Yogurt recipes: Greek Yogurt Pancakes, Salad with Greek Yogurt Dressing, Pasta in Greek Yogurt Sauce.

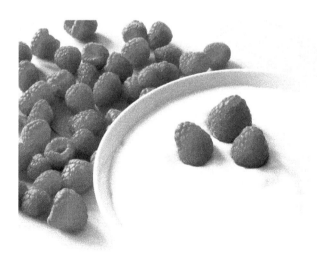

9. Tofu

Tofu, also known as bean curd. Just like cottage cheese, tofu is prepared by coagulating soy milk and then pressing the resulting curds into solid white blocks. Tofu is the richest source of protein as it contains all nine essential amino acids. It is also a valuable source of iron, calcium, copper, zinc, vitamin B1, phosphorous, manganese, and selenium.

100 grams of tofu contains 8 grams of protein.

Tofu recipes: Tofu Nuggets, Asian Garlic Tofu, Tofu Manchurian.

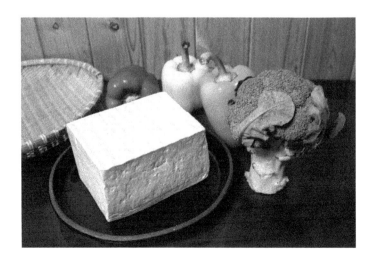

10. Green Peas

Peas are a complete protein, containing all nine essential amino acids. Along with protein, peas have a high level of Vitamin K. In addition, peas are a good source of dietary fiber, Vitamin A, Vitamin C, iron, folate, thiamin, and manganese.

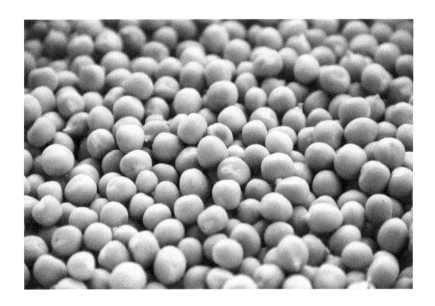

Both fresh and dried green peas are higher in protein. You can soak the dried green peas in plenty of water, overnight, or for 6-8 hours. Drain the soaking water. Place this in a pressure cooker with 2 cups of fresh water. Pressure cook for 1 whistle. Now it is ready to use in your recipes.

100 grams of Peas contain 6 grams of protein.

Green Peas recipes: Green Peas Cutlet, Peas Fried Rice, Peas and Mint Soup.

My Thoughts

Protein is an important building block of bones, muscles, nails. Our body requires protein for repairing and making enzymes, hormones, and other chemicals of the body. Insufficient protein intake in vegetarians is not uncommon. The above listed protein-rich foods are readily available in the market and one can easily include them in their diet

4 10 Healthy Carbohydrates You Must Eat For Health And Nutrition Benefits

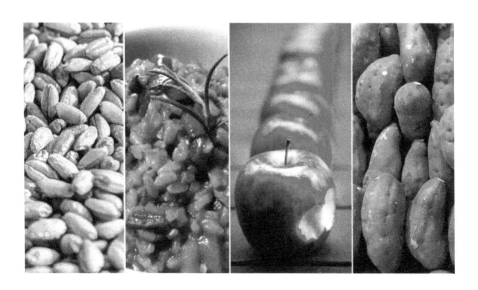

10 Healthy Carbohydrates You Must Eat For Health And Nutrition Benefits

What are Carbs/Carbohydrates?

Carbohydrates are one of three macronutrients — along with proteins and fats — that your body requires daily.

Simple carbohydrates are carbohydrates that contain single monosaccharide units. They are broken down quickly by the body to be used as energy. They are found in natural food sources such as milk, milk products, fruit, and vegetables.

Complex carbohydrates are polysaccharides which are made up of complex chains of thousands of monosaccharide units. Complex carbohydrates digest slowly and take time to absorb to the body. They are found in whole grains, legumes, and starchy vegetables, like potatoes.

Why carbs are important?

The main function of carbohydrates is to provide the body and brain with energy. Carbohydrates improve brain power, reduce cancer risk, improve digestion and sleep pattern.

Below is the list of 10 High-Quality Carbohydrates that you must eat for Health and Nutrition Benefits:

1. Whole Wheat

Unlike unhealthy Refined wheat which is processed to remove the bran and the germ, leaving only the endosperm, whole-wheat is made from the entire wheat kernels—bran, germ, and endosperm which makes them highly nutritious.

Gluten is a group of proteins, occur with starch in the endosperm of wheat, as refined wheat or white flour only consist of endosperm, gluten is quite high in them. Amount of gluten present in 3 cups of whole wheat flour is equivalent to the amount of gluten present in 1 cup of white flour.

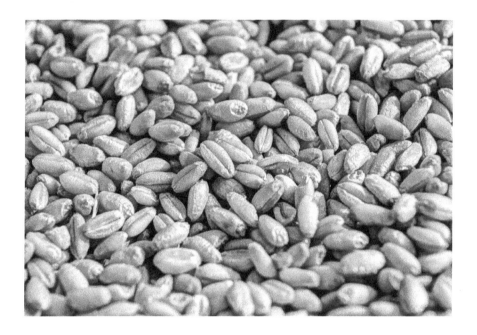

Whole wheat is a rich source of vitamin B6, dietary fiber, iron, calcium, potassium, magnesium, etc. Whole wheat has plenty of complex carbohydrates which give sustained energy. Bran from whole wheat provides dietary fiber which helps in reducing blood cholesterol levels and may lower risk of heart disease.

100 g of Whole wheat flour contains 72 g of total carbohydrates, of which 11 g is dietary fiber.

2. Brown Rice

Brown rice is whole-grain rice from which only inedible the husk (the outermost layer) is removed while from white rice, along with the hull, the bran layer and the germ (the next layers underneath the husk) are also removed, leaving mostly the starchy endosperm. Several vitamins and dietary minerals are lost in this removal and the further polishing process.

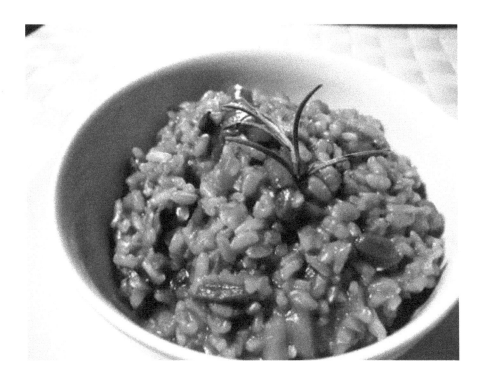

Brown rice is a good source of vitamin B1, B2, B6, magnesium, selenium, phosphorus, and is high in fiber. Brown rice is considered a low glycemic index food as it digests more slowly, causing a lower change in blood sugar level. The soluble fiber in brown rice attaches to cholesterol particles and takes them out of the body, helping to reduce overall cholesterol levels and may help prevent the formation of blood clots.

100 g of raw brown rice contains 73 g of total carbohydrate, of which 3.52 g is dietary fiber.

3. Oats

Oat groats are the whole form of oats, these are mostly intact, hulled oat grains. Groats include the cereal germ and fiber-rich bran portion of the grain, as well as the endosperm.

For steel cuts oats, oats groats are processed by chopping the whole oat groat into several pieces. For rolled oats, oats groats are first steamed to make them soft, then pressed to flatten them. For instant oats, oats groats pre-cooked, dried, and then pressed slightly thinner than rolled oats.

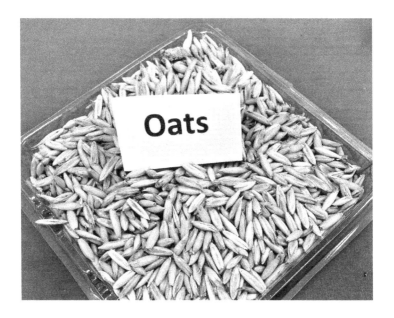

Steel cuts oats are slightly higher in fiber than rolled while Instant oats are the most highly processed variety and have quite less nutritional value. Oat groats are the healthiest among all types of oats. You can coarsely grind oat groats into flour and use this flour in making bread, cookies, and chapattis.

Oats are gluten-free whole grain and an excellent source of protein, dietary fiber, antioxidants, vitamins, and minerals, especially manganese.

Oat is a rich source of the water-soluble fiber β-glucan which help keep cholesterol in check, may help manage diabetes. Oats promote healthy bacteria in the digestive tract, help fight cardiovascular disease, and Type 2 diabetes.

100 g of oats contain 66.3 g of total carbohydrate, of which 11g is dietary fiber, 4 g of soluble fiber β-glucan.

4. Quinoa

Quinoa is a seed-producing flowering plant. It is pseudocereal which means unlike wheat and rice, quinoa is not a grass but are used in much the same way as cereals. Quinoa seed can be ground into flour and otherwise used as cereals.

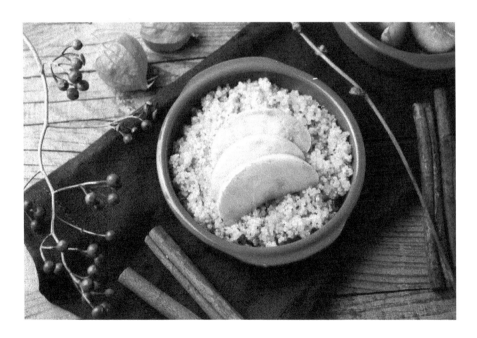

Quinoa is high in complex carbohydrate, insoluble fiber, and protein which makes it very filling. It has complete protein, means it contains all nine essential amino acids. It is also high in iron, magnesium, calcium, potassium, B vitamins, vitamin E, phosphorus, vitamin E and antioxidants.

Another good part is quinoa is gluten-free, so people with gluten intolerance can eat quinoa to meet their daily recommended carbs requirement.

Quinoa has the anti-inflammatory property, regulate body temperature, aids enzyme activity.

100 g of raw quinoa contains 64.2 g of complex carbohydrate, of which 7 g is dietary fiber.

5. Sweet Potatoes

Sweet potatoes are a rich source of fiber as well as containing an array of vitamins and minerals including iron, calcium, selenium, and they're a good source of most of our B vitamins and vitamin C. One of the key nutritional benefits of sweet potatoes are that they're high in an antioxidant known as beta-carotene, which converts to vitamin A once consumed.

Raw sweet potatoes are rich in complex carbohydrates and are a rich source of dietary fiber as well as containing an array of vitamins such as B vitamins and vitamin C, moderately contain vitamin B5, vitamin B6, and minerals including iron, calcium, selenium, manganese. One of the key nutritional benefits of sweet potatoes are that they're high in beta-carotene, an antioxidant which converts to vitamin A once consumed in the body.

Sweet potatoes protect the body from free radicals

protects against cancer, Support Immune System, Support Healthy Vision.

100 g of sweet potatoes contain 20 g of complex carbohydrate, of which 3 g is dietary fiber.

6. Boiled Potatoes

Boiled potatoes have a lower glycemic score than naked baked potatoes. Because of the lower glycemic score, our body digest boiled potatoes more slowly make them easier to digest and keep us feeling full longer.

Boiled potatoes cooked with skin are very low in Saturated Fat, Sodium, contain zero cholesterol.

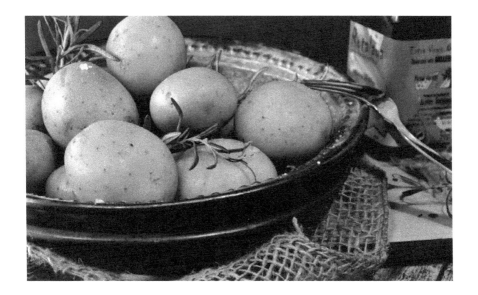

A large, unpeeled boiled potato is rich in B-complex vitamins. A boiled potato provides more than half of the recommended daily intake of vitamin B6. It is also a good source of, Potassium and Copper, and a very good source of Vitamin C.

It contains resistant Starch that improves Gut health by making more good bacteria and less bad bacteria in the gut. Moreover, boiled potatoes are gluten-free.

100 g of boiled potatoes contain 20 g of total carbohydrate, of which 1.6 g is dietary fiber.

7. Apples

For the greatest health benefits, eat the whole apple - both skin and flesh. Apples are extremely rich in dietary fiber. The soluble fiber content of apples may promote weight loss and gut health.

1 medium-sized apple contains 95 calories, it takes 150 calories to digest an apple. It means you will burn an additional 50 calories simply by eating an apple.

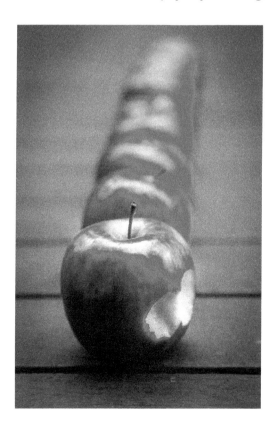

Apples are highly rich in important antioxidants, flavonoids. The phytonutrients and antioxidants in apples may help reduce the risk of developing diabetes, hypertension, heart disease, and cancer.

Other health benefits of apples include prevention of stomach, and liver disorders, anemia, gallstones, and constipation.

100 g of apples contain 14 g of total carbohydrate, of which 2.4 g is dietary fiber.

8. Bananas

Bananas are high in potassium, that promotes heart health. Eating them could help lower blood pressure and reduce the risks of cancer and asthma. Bananas are rich in fiber, calcium, vitamin B6, vitamin C, and various antioxidants and phytonutrients. Unripe bananas have a high content of resistant starch which promotes intestinal health.

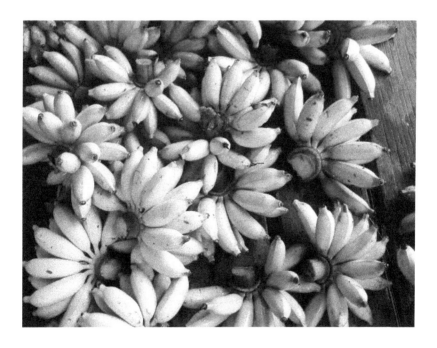

Bananas have a low glycemic index. Due to the high iron content, bananas are good for those suffering from anemia. Bananas have a decent amount of magnesium, which has been known to aid sound sleep.

100 g of bananas contain 23 g of total carbohydrate, of which 2.6 g is dietary fiber.

9. Chickpeas

Chickpeas are high in complex carbohydrates which make you feel full for a longer period of time as they digest slowly. The starch found in chickpeas is digested slowly and supports more stabilized blood sugar levels. Chickpeas are high in protein which helps in weight loss. The fiber in chickpeas absorb water and attach to toxins and waste as they move through the digestive system, forming stool, which contains toxins and waste that must be removed from the body.

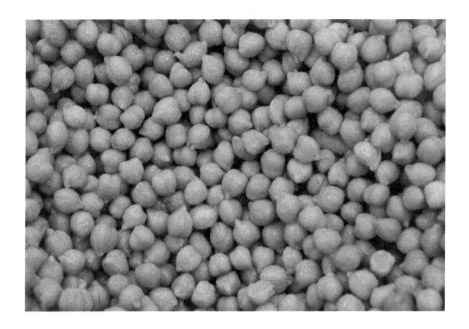

They are a rich source of the essential vitamin B complex (B1, B2, B3 B6, B12), vitamin A, vitamin C, and vitamin K, antioxidants and minerals such as iron, magnesium, zinc, phosphorous and folate.

100 g of chickpeas contain 61 g of total carbohydrate, of which 17 g is dietary fiber.

10. Kidney Beans

Kidney beans contain both soluble and insoluble fiber, which keep your digestive system running smoothly. Soluble fiber can bind cholesterol in the intestine and remove it from the body and insoluble fiber adds bulk to the stool and helps prevent constipation.

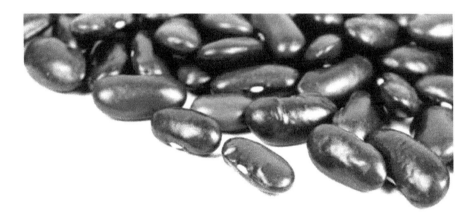

They contain slow carbohydrates which means the carbohydrates break down and are absorbed from the intestines slowly avoiding sudden blood sugar spikes. Antioxidants found in kidney beans help combat cancer. Additionally, calcium and magnesium in kidney beans can prevent osteoporosis and strengthen the bones. Kidney beans are among the richest sources of plant-based protein which boost muscle mass.

100 g of kidney beans contain 6 g of total carbohydrate, of which 25 g is dietary fiber.

Conclusion

Health benefits of high-quality carbohydrates rich food are countless. Don't confuse healthy carbs with refined processed carbs such as cookies, donuts. To meet recommended daily carbs need one should never depend upon refined carbs. Add high-quality carbohydrates into your diet for a healthy life. Carbohydrate-restricted diets possess possible risks of osteoporosis and cancer incidence. But one should keep this in mind that eating carbs in excess may result in weight gain.

5 10 Power Foods To Eat To Get Rid Of Anemia

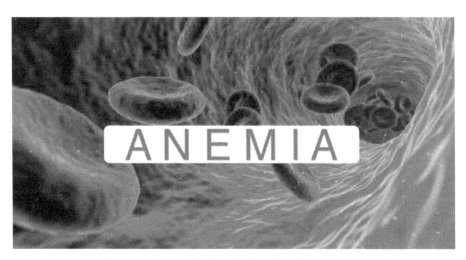

10 Power Foods To Eat To Get Rid Of Anemia

What is Anemia?

Iron Deficiency Anemia is a common type of Anemia- a condition in which there is a deficiency of red cells or of hemoglobin in the blood.

As the name implies iron deficiency anemia is due to insufficient iron in the body. Without enough iron, body can't produce enough of hemoglobin in red blood cells. Hemoglobin is the main part of red blood cells and binds oxygen. Hemoglobin in the blood carries oxygen from the lungs or gills to the rest of the body.

Cause of Anemia

Iron deficiency is amongst the most common of nutritional deficiencies and the most common cause of anemia globally, although other conditions, such as folate, vitamin B12 and vitamin A deficiencies, can all cause anemia.

Inadequate iron intake due to poor diet, blood loss through heavy periods, inflammatory bowel disease and increased requirements during pregnancy lead to anemia.

Symptoms of Anemia

Iron deficiency anemia signs and symptoms may include:

- Fatigue
- Dizziness
- Cold hands and feet
- Weakness
- Pale skin
- Irregular heartbeats
- Shortness of breath, particularly with exercise

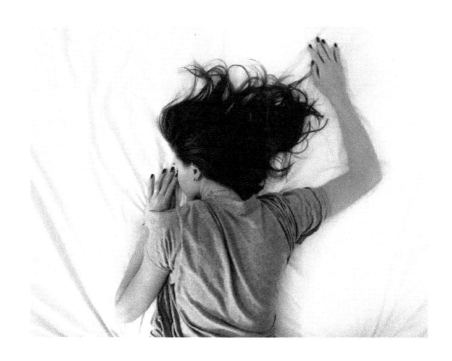

With proper diet, rich in iron one can get rid of anemia.

Heme Iron and Non-Heme Iron

The two forms of dietary iron are Heme Iron and Non-Heme Iron: Heme iron is the type of iron that comes from animal proteins like seafood, meat, poultry, and fish.

Iron from plants is known as non-heme iron and is found in plant-based foods like grains, fruits, beans, vegetables, fruits, nuts, and seeds and in iron-fortified foods such as oats.

Vitamin C helps your stomach absorb iron. Try to combine non-heme iron foods with vitamin C (for example, a glass of lemon juice, orange, berries, kiwi fruit, tomatoes, and capsicum) to increase absorption of iron.

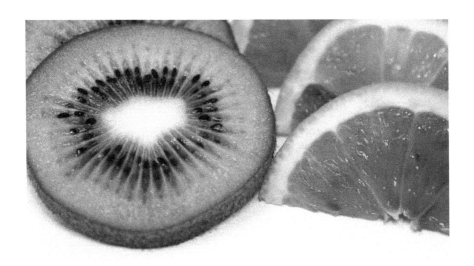

As this is a vegetarian zone we will discuss vegetarian options in detail.

Below is the List of 10 Power Foods To Eat To Get Rid Of Anemia:

1. Spinach

Spinach is rich in Iron, beta-carotene, calcium, vitamin B9 and C and fiber. Regular consumption of spinach can prevent anemia. Spinach is much better than red meat as it provides fewer calories and is fat and cholesterol free. To make the most of its health benefits, include spinach in your daily diet. Make sure to combine vitamin-C-rich foods such as citrus fruits with spinach to improve absorption.

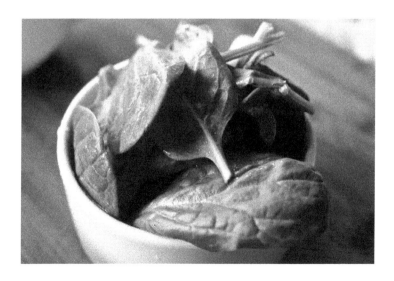

2. Beetroot

Beetroot is loaded with iron and vitamin C, which is considered good for anemia. Beetroot helps in repairing and reactivating the red blood cells in the body. Once activated, oxygen can easily be transferred to the muscles and other tissues of the body. Adding beetroot in any form in your daily diet will help to easily fight anemia.

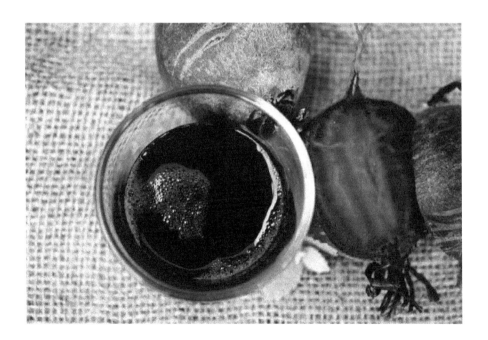

3. Lentils

Legumes—especially lentils—are great for anemia, as just a half-cup has around 20% of iron what your body needs for the day. Legumes are also high in folate, magnesium, potassium, and fiber that fills you up may help lower cholesterol and may help stabilize your blood sugar and may even aid weight loss.

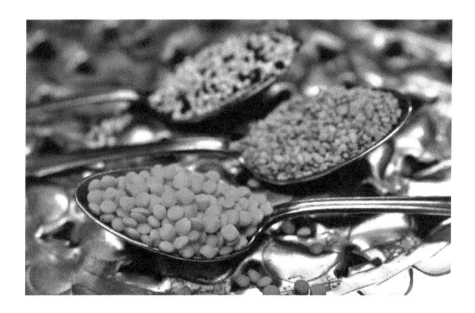

4. Honey

Honey is among the most popular and widely used sweetener with enormous health benefits. Honey is a rich source of iron. Along with Iron, copper, and magnesium in honey increase hemoglobin concentration in your blood, thereby treating anemia. Adding one tablespoon of honey to a glass of lukewarm water with some lemon juice early in the morning on an empty stomach every day will help in effectively fighting anemia.

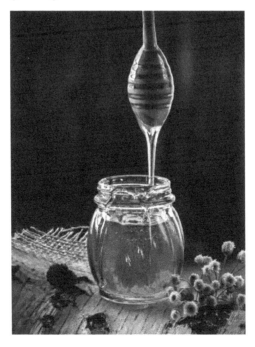

5. Jaggery/ Panela

Jaggery is commonly known as *gur* in India and panela in the rest of the world. Regular intake of jaggery in any form with any food will help combat anemia. Jaggery is unrefined sugar, in fact, it is the purest form of sugar and is prepared in iron vessels with fruit juices without any addition of synthetic chemicals. It is rich in iron and folate which help prevent anemia. Regular intake of jaggery with ginger juice helps in better absorption of iron.

6. Chickpeas

Chickpeas are Iron powerhouse for vegetarians. Chickpeas are high in fiber and protein and contain several key vitamins and minerals. They are rich in iron, folate and vitamin C, which are necessary for the synthesis of hemoglobin. Higher protein and iron content of chickpeas, make them a smart option for vegetarians. Add lemon juice to hummus for better iron absorption.

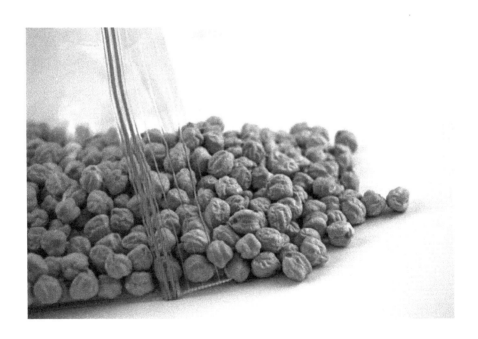

7. Pumpkin Seeds

Pumpkin seeds are rich in iron, antioxidants, zinc, magnesium and many other nutrients. Only a handful of pumpkin seeds every two days can help strengthen the immune system, prevent anemia. Add the roasted pumpkin seeds to morning cereal, bread, yogurt, or salad topping.

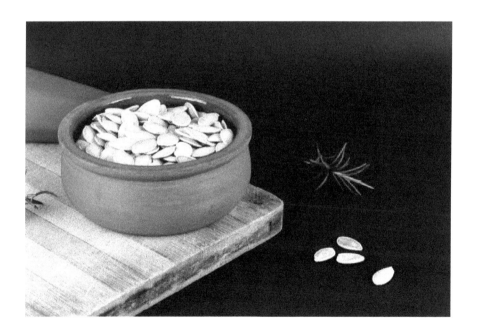

8. Fenugreek

The fenugreek seeds rich in proteins with essential amino acids, Iron, Ascorbate and Folate content, have restorative and nutritive properties. Fenugreek helps to prevent and cure anemia and maintain a good healthy life for a longer duration. The leaves of fenugreek help in blood formation. The seeds of fenugreek are also a valuable cure for anemia being rich in iron.

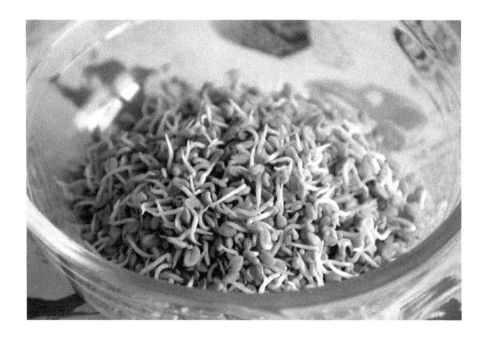

9. Soybeans

Soybeans are a major source of non-heme iron. Soybean is low in fat and high in protein and fiber that fights anemia. They're an excellent source of important minerals like copper, which helps keep our blood vessels and immune system healthy. It is also high in manganese, an essential nutrient involved in many chemical processes in the body.

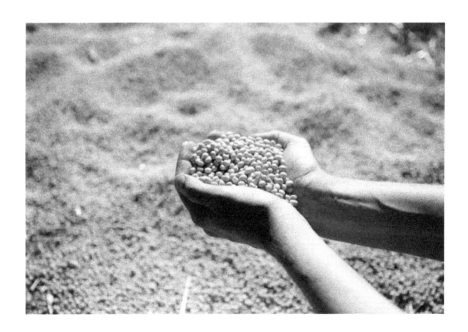

10. Sesame Seeds

The iron in sesame seeds can keep the immune system functioning properly and prevent iron-deficient anemia. Especially the black sesame seeds are a rich source of iron. The seeds are packed with essential nutrients, like copper, phosphorus, vitamin E, and zinc as well. One quarter cup size serving of sesame seeds can provide 30% of the daily iron requirement.

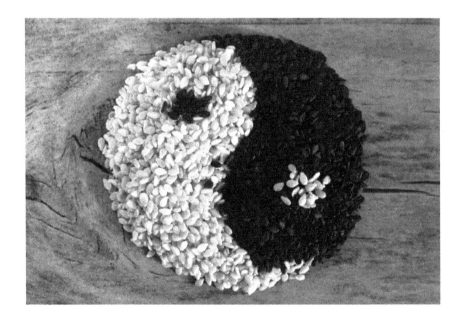

Conclusion

Body cannot produce iron on its own which is an important mineral, it plays a key role in cell growth and differentiation, therefore, consuming Iron rich diet on a regular basis is important. Remember to include a source of vitamin C when eating non-heme plant sources of iron to boost its absorption in the body. Girls should increase iron consumption during periods to combat the blood loss, similarly women who are pregnant should increase the iron consumption as they are at a higher risk for developing anemia due to the excess amount of blood the body produces to help provide nutrients for the baby

About the Author

La Fonceur is a Dance Artist and a Health Blogger. La Fonceur is Masters in Pharmacy specialized in Pharmaceutical Technology. She has published a Review Article on "Techniques for Producing Biotechnology-Derived Products of Pharmaceutical Use" in Pharmtechmedica Journal. She is a Registered State Pharmacist. She is National Level GPAT Qualifier in the year 2011 and among Top 1400 nationwide. Being a Research Scientist, she has worked closely with drugs and based on her experience she believes Vegetarian Foods are the remedy for many diseases, one can prevent most of the diseases with Nutritional Foods and Healthy Lifestyle.

CPSIA information can be obtained
at www.ICGtesting.com
Printed in the USA
BVHW091135240223
659163BV00015B/891